OXFORD MEDICAL PUBLICATIONS

On-Call

PRACTICAL GUIDES FOR GENERAL PRACTICE

1. *Cervical screening: a practical guide*
   Ann McPherson
2. *A basic formulary for general practice*
   G. B. Grant, D. A. Gregory, and T. D. van Zwanenberg
3. *Radiology*
   Robert F. Bury
4. *Stroke*
   Derick Wade
5. *Alcohol*
   P. Anderson
6. *Breast cancer screening*
   Joan Austoker and John Humphreys
7. *Computers: a guide to choosing and using*
   Tom Stewart and Andrew Willis
8. *Immunizing children*
   Sue Sefi and J. A. Macfarlane
9. *On-Call: out-of-hours telephone calls and home visits*
   J. D. E. Knox
10. *Breast cancer screening* (Scottish edition)
    Joan Austoker and John Humphreys
11. *Screening tests used in children*
    J. A. Macfarlane, Sue Sefi, and M. Cordeiro

Forthcoming

Non-insulin-dependent diabetes
Ann-Louise Kinmonth

On-Call

Out-of-Hours Telephone Calls and Home Visits

Practical Guides for General Practice 9

J. D. E. KNOX

Professor of General Practice
University of Dundee

Oxford New York Tokyo
OXFORD UNIVERSITY PRESS
1989

Oxford University Press, Walton Street, Oxford OX2 6DP
Oxford New York Toronto
Delhi Bombay Calcutta Madras Karachi
Petaling Jaya Singapore Hong Kong Tokyo
Nairobi Dar es Salaam Cape Town
Melbourne Auckland

and associated companies in
Berlin Ibadan

Oxford is a trade mark of Oxford University Press

Published in the United States
by Oxford University Press, New York

British Library Cataloguing in Publication Data
Knox, J. D. E. (James D. E.)
On-call: out-of-hours telephone calls and
home visits.—(Practical guides for general
practice; 9
1. Great Britain. General practice.
Workloads
I. Title II. Series
362.1'72'0941
ISBN 0–19–261777–X

Library of Congress Cataloging in Publication Data
Knox, James D. E.
On-call: out-of-hours telephone calls and home visits/J.D.E.
Knox.
(Practical guide for general practice) (Oxford
medical publications)
Bibliography: Includes index.
1. Family medicine. 2. Visiting the sick. 3. Communication in
medicine. I. Title. II. Series. III. Series: Oxford medical
publications.
RC48.K66 1989 610.69'52—dc20 89-3408
ISBN 0–19–261777–X (pbk.)

Typeset by Cotswold Typesetting Ltd, Cheltenham
Printed by Dotesios Printers Limited
Trowbridge, Wiltshire.

To my wife and family

Preface

The practice of medicine has always involved work during 'unsocial hours'. This aspect of family medicine is a particularly emotive one, because of a potential clash of interests—on the one hand, a professional wish (and requirement) to be available and accessible to patients in their hour of need, and, on the other, the doctor's personal rights as an individual. The situation is intensified for the general practitioner because there is no clear career structure: delegation to a junior is not an option so readily available to the principal in NHS practice as it is to his hospital consultant colleague.

The medical profession has been concerned to evaluate the necessity for this generally unpopular component of workload. An increasingly consumer-orientated society has also made contributions to the literature, mainly on the theme of quality of the services to the patient. This book attempts to bring together these elements and combine them with an in-depth analysis of matters of clinical concern. The book is intended to help trainee general practitioners and new entrants to general practice to react in a more informed way to pressures both from within the profession and from outside it which are driving British general practice towards a '9 to 5' approach to patient care. The book will have achieved its objective if it promotes, especially in the training arena, a constructive debate on some of the complex issues involved.

Dundee   J. D. E. K.
January 1989

Acknowledgements

I am indebted to Dr A. Jacob, Dr J. Fletcher, Dr R. Neville, Dr P. Owen, Dr J. A. R. Lawson, and Professor J. Howie for reading early drafts of this work and for their useful suggestions, to Philip Smith for assistance with proof-reading, to Mrs A. Moss for typing successive drafts, and to the publishers for their patient help.

Dundee   J. D. E. K.
January 1989

Contents

1 Setting the scene

We were just visiting gran, whom we haven't seen for some time. We didn't like the look of her and thought it was time she had a thorough check-up.
— *Relatives who called out the general practitioner on a Sunday afternoon*

Her earache was so bad I had to call the doctor in the middle of the night. He was ages in coming. He wasn't our own GP—and I could hardly understand his accent. Next time I'll take her straight to Casualty...
— *Parent reporting experience with a deputizing service*

Police Constable Brown speaking. We've had to break into Mr McDonald's house; he's been found in a collapsed state. Will you come, please?
— *Urgent call on a Sunday night*

I don't want to bother you. Could you please advise me about my niece's baby—she's been crying since 8 o'clock.
— *Anxious baby-sitter at midnight*

I need my prescription for another Salbutamol inhaler.
— *Psychiatrically disturbed young adult phoning at 11 p.m.*

Aims and scope of the book

Because undergraduate medical education is based on hospital medicine, students have limited opportunities to learn about primary medical care. University Departments of General Practice have so much to teach in the curricular time available to them that out-of-hours work tends to be given a relatively low priority, quite apart from the practical difficulties of involving the student in this aspect of care. For most entrants to general practice the first real experience of out-of-hours work comes during vocational training, and even then opportunities are often constrained by such factors as the development of rotas, reducing further the already limited number of times a practice will be 'on call' in the 'Trainee Year'.

This book is written as an adjunct to training, and it is therefore intended for use by both trainer and trainee. It aims to bring together information from both medical *and non-medical* sources to assist the trainee to develop professional skills in a sensitive area of clinical practice. It discusses both out-of-hours requests and options open to the doctor in responding.

So what's the problem?

An important characteristic of general practice is the first-contact nature of the relationship between patients and doctor—this is why one of the terms used to describe UK general practice is 'primary care'. When this first contact is examined more closely, however, it becomes evident that in fact the person with whom the patient actually makes first contact is the receptionist, at least during normal working hours. The medium through which that contact is made in over half the contacts is the telephone.

Outside normal working hours, however, the picture is rather different. For a start, virtually *all* contacts which patients initially make with doctors are mediated through the telephone. Secondly, the contact, when it is made, connects the caller more directly with the doctor. Other important characteristics of out-of-hours calls are discussed more fully later, but already two important issues have been introduced, namely the telephone availability (and accessibility) of the doctor out-of-hours, and the business of telephone communications themselves. Handling the telephone call is as important as handling the consultation, 'yet telephone communication remains haphazard, undocumented and subject to the idiosyncrasies of individual practitioners'.[1] There is evidently room for improvement in the ways we, as general practitioners, manage a part of clinical medicine to which undergraduate education and postgraduate training appear to have paid scant attention.

Out-of-hours availability and accessibility of the doctor are matters about which few of us in general practice can be complacent. The General Medical Services Committee was sufficiently concerned to set up a working party to consider the issues and to prepare a code of practice.[2] Failure to meet appropriate standards without good reason carries with it a threat of disciplinary action from within the profession.

The three UK medical defence organizations all single out weakening doctor–patient relationships for special mention when discussing the rising tide of litigation against doctors, and the substantial increase in subscriptions in the last five years.

There is evidence[3] that patients are ever more willing to question and criticize their doctors and are generally more knowledgeable and self-confident about health matters: this trend is likely to continue. Consumer reaction to telephone access to general practitioners suggests that this is a subject of concern.[4]

Telephone technology continues to make rapid advances, yet doubts have been expressed[1] on the ability of such advances to come to grips with the more fundamental problems of telephone ownership for disadvantaged sections of society. Privatization of British Telecom (BT) may be associated with increasing commercial pressures to cut losses, and figures indicate that in 1984 public coin-boxes were operated at a loss of approximately £1000 per call-box per year. Unserviceability of public equipment for whatever reason—failure to accept money and vandalism are among the commonest reasons—add to the problems facing some patients—and doctors. BT have plans to reduce the current relatively high rate of unserviceable public telephones (estimated nationally at about 25 per cent,[5] but much higher in certain localities).

It is evident that telephone access and communication between doctor and patient, especially out of hours, present many complex issues. To simplify matters, and provide doctors with a coherent account on which they may make more informed decisions, this booklet has deliberately focused attention on the out-of-hours dimension, using an approach based on the practicalities of patient care.

The out-of-hours dimension

Out-of-hours calls have a number of features which set them apart from other calls. It is the doctor (or his phone-sitter— often a member of his family), rather than the receptionist who deals with the call. Out-of-hours calls are more likely to be concerned with clinical matters, and less with appointments and repeat prescriptions. Usually the message (at least for the UK general practitioner) is a request for a home visit: with most such requests, it is not the patient who makes the call, but a third party. Furthermore, the clinical probabilities of out-of-hours health problems are different. Nighttime is associated with a number of specific clinical entities (such as paroxysmal *nocturnal* dyspnoea and croup in children) as well as a number of more general features (such as an increase in pyrexia, a worsening of confusion in the elderly, and a heightening of levels of anxiety). Increased levels of anxiety may influence assessment of the urgency of a situation by the lay observer. In addition to the above, cover for out-of-hours calls involves the doctor and his household in work during 'unsocial hours', interfering with sleep and recreation, a fact recognized by the National Health Service in the additional item-of-service payments under the appropriate regulations. Over and above these features of out-of-hours requests, telephone calls have characteristics which set them apart from other forms of communication in medicine.

Telephone communications: constraints and opportunities

Constraints

Among the more obvious constraints is the time factor, which may be accentuated in the call from a coin-operated public call-box. There is the loss of the non-verbal mode of communication, a normal accompaniment of direct speech; this loss may be compensated for in a number of ways, but these may themselves distort the message. An associated loss of the availability of objective physical findings is one reason why some doctors consider it almost impossible without a visit to give patients sensible and safe advice—a further factor which adds to stress experienced by doctors. Another consideration is the more limited control the doctor has both in directing the flow of conversation and of the decision-making environment. Some of this lack is associated with the indirect nature of the contact with the patient, since studies show that the caller is twice as likely to be a relative or 'significant other person' as a patient himself. These and other constraints are particularly important because the content of telephone conversations often has a larger element of negotiation between the parties than has face-to-face communication. Another characteristic of medical telephone communications is the relatively free nature of the emotional component, which may sometimes be amazingly uninhibited.[6]

Despite the wider availability of private telephones in the UK (some three-quarters of households now have a telephone, compared to under one-third in the 1950s) some callers are unfamiliar with the instrument and its use as a mode of communication. One indication of unfamiliarity with the use of the telephone is the duration of the 'pips' before the caller from a coin-operated phone makes contact. It has been suggested[7] that the longer the duration of the pips the greater will be the task facing the doctor in deciphering the message!

The caller may also be unaware of the practice's arrangements for out-of-hours cover,[8] and may be confused by them.

Some advantages

On the other hand, communication by telephone has a number of advantages for doctor and patient alike. For the patient, in addition to a ready means for summoning help, it can afford much-needed reassurance not simply in the nature of the professional advice given but in the knowledge that such advice and support may be readily available. Part of the success of the telephone Samaritans, 'Nite-line', and other agencies lies in this availability, coupled with the medium's suitability for the transmission of emotionally-laden messages.

A relatively recent development has been the wider availability to people of telephone professional advice on health matters through agencies such as Healthcall, which offer a 24-hours service.[9] Most such services rely on taped messages, but some are manned by volunteers: one example is Cry-sis, aimed at mothers worried about persistently crying babies. These services operate apart from general practice.

Some general practitioners set aside a specified time during working hours when they make themselves available to their patients for telephone discussions. This development, and other ways of working in the practice during normal office hours, may decrease the volume and alter the nature of out-of-hours calls.

For the doctror who wishes to use it as a convenient means of follow-up, the telephone can contribute to reducing the visiting load: however, such usages may alter significantly the way some patients seek help, and this factor may need to be taken into consideration when a new doctor is providing out-of-hours cover for a different practice, and when a practice is being taken over by a new doctor.

Some definitions

So far the word 'call' has been used in two different senses—a request for help (a telephone call), and also one of the options open to the doctor in responding to the request (a house call). This distinction is often not clearly made in the literature, much of which appears to be more concerned with doctors' out-of-hours visits; and this ambiguity may account, in part, for the widely differing rates of out-of-hours calls reported by general practitioners.

Failure to include *all* incoming telephone calls in calculating rates appears to have under-represented the extent to which UK doctors have in fact been using telephone advice in the past.[10] This booklet deals with *both* out-of-hours telephone calls *and* home visits: where appropriate, the meaning will be made clear by referring to the telephone call as a 'request' and the doctor's response as a 'visit'.

Urgency (see p. 31) refers to the speed which is called for in dealing with a given situation; emergency is an unforeseen occurrence or combination of circumstances calling for immediate action or remedy. There are two aspects to such assessments, lay (expressed in 'demand') and professional (which defines 'need'): the two are sometimes widely different, and agreement on this issue may need to be negotiated. The contact between caller and doctor may turn into a consultation, sometimes termed indirect to distinguish it from face-to-face contact: the term 'indirect consultation' may also denote consultation through a third party (intermediary).

Out-of-hours refers to periods outside those usually covered by a receptionist: broadly speaking 6 p.m. to 8 a.m. the following morning during full working days, from mid-day on Saturday until the following Monday morning, and throughout the full duration of public holidays.

The term 'night call' is sometimes used to denote a request received and answered by a visit during the period 11 p.m. to 7 a.m., because such an item attracts an extra payment which the doctor may claim from the appropriate NHS authority.

A practical approach to the subject

Training in telephone decision-making has been suggested as a legitimate subject to be included in the basic training of all doctors.[11] However, attempts to do this have raised a number of problems. One report,[12] based on simulated patients making out-of-hours calls to general practitioners in America, concluded that teaching could not be didactic and prescriptive. A model based on thoroughness, logic, and consistency did not prove adequate for a situation in which experienced doctors exhibited so wide a range of unpredictable and yet adaptive and efficient behaviours!

With these constraints in mind, this book has been written to take some account of the following:

- illness;
- patient;
- doctor;
- family and context; and
- organization.

References

1. Allsop, J. and May, A. (1985). *Telephone access to GPs. A study of London*, Project Paper No. 53. King Edward's Hospital Fund, London.
2. General Medical Services Committee (1984). *Report of the GMSC working party on telephone answering services.* British Medical Association, London.
3. Jones, L., Leneman, L., and Maclean, U. (1987). In *Consumer feedback for the NHS: a literature review,* p. 30. King Edward's Hospital Fund, London.
4. Sawyer, L. and Arber, S. (1982). Changes in home visiting and night and weekend cover: the patient's view. *Brit. Med. J.* **284**, 1531–4.
5. Oftel survey (1988). Improvements disappoint despite BT bid for payphone perfection. *Dundee Courier and Advertiser,* 8 January.
6. Samuel, O. (1983). What annoys me most: the telephone. *Brit. Med. J.* **287**, 1599–1600.
7. Moulds, A., Martin, P., Martin, M., and Moulds, N. (1985). In *A handbook for the doctor's spouse,* p. 15. Medical Sciences Liaison Division, Upjohn.
8. Cartwright, A. and Anderson, R. (1981). *General practice revisited: a second study of patients and their doctors.* Routledge & Kegan Paul, London.
9. Bryan, J. (1988). Help that is just a phone call away. *Independent,* 5th January.
10. Coleman, N. S. (1987). Telephone advice in managing out-of-hours calls. *J. Roy. Coll. Gen. Pract.* **37**, 463.
11. British Medical Journal (1978). Leading article. The telephone in general practice. *Brit. Med. J.* **2**, 1106.
12. Sloane, P. D., Egelhoff, C., Curtis, P., *et al.* (1985). Physician decision making over the telephone. *J. Family Practice,* **21**, 279–84.

2 Organization and equipment

Because the telephone is *the* medium through which out-of-hours contact is made between patient and doctor, transfer of calls from the surgery is central to a discussion on organization of on-call cover. The rate of progress of telephone technology (including miniaturization and increased portability of equipment), variations in costs over time (equipment is becoming cheaper), and widely differing local circumstances (including geography), all place constraints on discussion, so that only broad statements can be made. Detailed information should be sought from local telephone managers and the Primary Care Administrator.

Message-taking out of hours

In addition to the time-honoured single line extension to the doctor's home, a number of options are now available, including the following:

- Telephone answering machines.
- Subscriber controlled transfer.
- Customer call forwarding and commercial answering services.
- Change number intercept.
- Star and X-services.

In addition to such external services, some group practices employ a resident caretaker, who may combine a variety of practice duties with living on the premises: these staff take all incoming out-of-hours telephone messages and verbally relay them to the duty doctor, via ordinary telephone lines or radiopager. Such a system at least ensures for the patient a human (as opposed to mechanical) response to the caller, who is required to make only *one* telephone call. A possible disadvantage is that the option of negotiation with the caller and telephone advice become less available: the result is to increase the likelihood that the doctor has to visit.

Telephone answering machines are now relatively cheap: equipment can be purchased for as little as £80 (1988 prices)—see Appendix 3.

The machine may be a simple tape-recording without a reception facility. It usually plays a message, repeated once, such as 'The surgery is now closed until 8 a.m. In case of emergency ring Dr X at .... [appropriate telephone number]). Most recording machines allow space for receiving a message, and equipment is now available to provide remote playback so that the doctor, as he moves around, can check for urgent messages left on equipment at the surgery. The receiving facility does not appear to be widely used by general practitioners, because initiative to access the recorded information lies with the doctor, and some requests require an immediate response. There is an answering machine which also pages the doctor when a message is received.

There is no question that the advent of the answering machine has increased the flexibility of on-call arrangements. However, this advantage to the doctor may be at the expense of the caller, who usually has to make a second call to establish contact. Patients may perceive the answering machine as a barrier; some doctors deliberately to add to the barrier image by messages such as 'The surgery is now closed. Only if your call is an emergency, I repeat, only if your call is an emergency, dial ....'. Experience with the answering tapes produced by doctors suggests that there is room for improvement in the quality of recording, the rate of delivery, and the nature of the messages.

Subscriber controlled transfer (SCT) is a system whereby

incoming calls to the surgery on one or more numbers may automatically be re-routed to an external number on the same exchange. It is up to the practice staff going off duty to make the necessary diversion, and human as well as technical errors can occur in this system. Customer call forwarding (CCF) allows incoming calls to be intercepted and automatically diverted to a wider range of numbers than SCT (see below).

Change number intercept (CNI) is a service controlled by a telephone exchange operator. The doctor can initiate this diversion service by calling 'intercept' from any telephone, and instructing the exchange to intercept calls on one or more numbers, and, verbally, advise the caller to dial the number of the doctor on call. The advantage to the patient of being able to converse with a human being is off-set by the lack of immediacy in obtaining an appropriate medical response—a further telephone call is needed. On occasion this service may also be so slow to answer the ringing tone as to lead the caller to believe the doctor's telephone to be unattended.

More up-to-date technology allows the doctor to divert calls by tapping out a sequence of numbers on appropriate equipment: BT's Star and X services are examples. Call diversions can be of several kinds: the most relevant to the doctor are 'basic diversion', which diverts all incoming calls to another number, and 'diversion on no reply', which diverts incoming calls to another number if the phone is not picked up within 15 seconds. This latter diversion, coupled to a taped answering machine, allows the caller to get through without having to make a second call: the cost of the diverted call, however, is now borne by the practice. Star services afford a wide range of other telephone activities, some of which are more relevant to general practice work during 'office hours'.

A number of commercial telephone answering services are available to general practitioners. Medical Answerline, for example, provides a round-the-clock personal answering service, whereby incoming calls are automatically re-directed to the Answerline receptionist. The message can then be dealt with in one of a variety of ways. It can be phoned in to Air Call (a commercial deputizing service), or directed to the subscribing doctor's nearest telephone, or the service may 'bleep' the doctor using a range of pagers, including transmission of voice or visual messages (see also the section on phone-sitting).

Alerting the doctor

In addition to the business of dealing with incoming tele-phone calls, there is the question of alerting the doctor when he is away from base. The widespread availability of tele-phones in patients' homes allows the phone-sitter to alert the doctor out on visits, provided the phone-sitter knows the route the doctor is likely to follow and the telephone number of the households being visited. There are other local (and sometimes idiosyncratic) ways of indicating to a doctor out on visits that another call has come in, such as switching on a flashing outside light at a branch surgery. Nowadays, how-ever, radiopagers of various kinds are in widespread use. They are of two main kinds, the on-site (the kind usually encountered in hospitals) and the national zone wide-ranging service.[1] This latter, more relevant to general practice, offers a number of options. There are pagers that bleep (tone and silent) and others which display visual messages (display page and message master). A more sophisticated development is the cellular radiophone for use in the car. Some more advanced equipment can be un-clipped and carried by the doctor as he goes into the patient's house. With each increasing level of sophistication the price of equipment rises, as does the cost of mainten-ance.

Maintenance of equipment

With increasing availability of equipment of all kinds on sale, the buyer may feel the need for guidance from those who have first-hand experience. There is also the question of maintenance. When something goes wrong, if there is no 'on-site' maintenance contract, the doctor may be deprived of the facility when the equipment is sent to a central depot for servicing—the failure may also incur a call-out fee. Some equipment, such as simple answering machines, is relatively cheap, so that it might be more economical to purchase a spare to cover failures. British Telecom provide a number of different maintenance contracts, the cost of which may be born by the NHS provided the equipment is approved by British Telecom: this might include, under certain circum- stances, some privately purchased equipment, but the doctor should first check the situation with the local tele- phone manager.

Organizing out-of-hours cover

Much of this booklet is based on the assumption that British general practice wishes to continue the 'extended system of care', because it is the compromise which maximizes personal and continuing care, in contradistinction to con- tinuity of care. Other possibilities exist, including deputizing services and a 'shift' approach to the problem. This last has long been accepted by the nursing profession—has it any- thing to offer UK general practice? Something approaching this system might result from moves being made in job sharing in practice.[2]

Extended cover

Within many group practices, the partners have an agree- ment to take in turn the provision of out-of-hours cover.

Patterns of out-of-hours incoming calls are too varied to make firm generalizations, but Friday nights tend to be unpopular with some doctors because the commitment to handing over next day encroaches on the weekend off-duty; in the case of a rota outside the practice the juxtaposition raises the possibility of one practice being responsible for an unduly prolonged period of cover. These and other matters are best dealth with by written agreements. With larger rotas, division of the out-of-hours load should take account of such factors as the numbers of partners (and other doctors), the size of the practice lists, and the workload associated with them, to ensure the workload is distributed fairly. In the week-to-week running of agreed arrangements, the practice manager is often well placed to supervise the system and to approach individual doctors when adjustments are necessitated by unforeseen circumstances.

Deputizing services

Deputizing services are now established and in widespread use, not simply restricted to single-handed practices and small groups. In one study, a quarter of practices using deputizing services were groups of four or more doctors.[3] The public may be somewhat resentful when doctors in large practices resort to using deputizing services, since they are well aware that one of the benefits of group practice is that partners should be able to provide out-of-hours cover for each other.[4] On the other hand, the realities of urban deprivation may combine to produce an intolerably high night-visiting rate: a burden which even an organized large group of doctors could not sustain without help from a deputizing service.[5] In circumstances which make it difficult for a patient to get a reasonable, good-humoured out-of-hours service, deputizing may be better for all concerned.[6] Such regular use, however, has wider implications. Frequent use deprives trainee general practitioners of essential experience; it also generates a feeling that such a way of working cuts across the personal caring traditions of British general practice. For these reasons, regular and repeated recourse to deputizing services now precludes a practice from appointment as a training practice in at least one region in Scotland.[7]

The extended lines of communication in deputizing services may afford greater opportunities for mistakes. When something goes seriously wrong with a deputizing service, not only is it often the case that a number of mistakes or delays have already occurred, but tempers may run high.[8]

A call to a deputizing service is very much more likely to result in a visit than is the case with rota systems (one study reports 97 per cent of requests to deputizing services resulting in a visit),[5] and the range of management options is narrowed.

Training considerations

Vocational training properly includes providing for the trainee *supervised* experience in out-of-hours calls. If the trainee lives within the area covered by the telephone exchange associated with the practice, the technical problems of re-routing the calls are simplified. If the trainee lives at a distance, consideration should be given to providing him with suitable accommodation to afford first-hand experience in handling incoming calls, should it prove impossible to re-direct them. It is the trainer's responsibility to finance the cost elements of telephone provision.

The trainer needs to exercise judgement on the readiness of the new trainees to 'go solo'. After two or three nights on call when both trainer and trainee make visits together it is usually possible to encourage the trainee to cope unaided, but with the trainer being readily available throughout the on-call period.

Phone-sitting

The contribution made by the doctor's spouse to ensuring continuing care of the patients in a practice over the years has not received the recognition it deserves. In recent years, the tradition that this task should automatically fall to the doctor's spouse is being increasingly called in question, even if it should be possible to pay a salary. An impetus towards putting 'on call' on a more business-like basis is provided by the increasing proportion of married women in general practice—women whose wage-earning husbands may not so readily accept a role which, in the past, has been passively assumed by wives and families.

Some easing of the pressures on the phone-sitter has resulted from advances in telephone technology ('customer call forwarding') in association with commercial telephone answering services. This should not be confused with deputizing services (see p. 15). Telephone answering services are employed by the subscribing doctor as a phone-sitting service in which a human agent will receive an incoming call and relay it to the doctor, usually by pager: such services merely take and relay messages, and it is unreasonable to expect them to make medical decisions.

The occasional use of such services is well received by the patients and doctors in one large rural practice covering a wide area in North East Scotland. The patient rings the practice number. By means of CCF the call is automatically relayed to a receiving centre some 40 miles distant. The caller is answered on a personalized line by an operator, who responds in the name of the practice. The receipt of the call is logged, and the duty-doctor is contacted by radio-pager. The doctor must acknowledge receipt of the call within fifteen minutes. If he fails to do this, a further attempt is made to contact him, which, if unsuccessful, may result in his colleague (whose number is available to the system) being contacted. The responsibility for the receipt of incoming calls remains with the subscriber (namely, the doctor).

Documentation

Most general practitioners record details of all incoming telephone calls, and later transfer selected information to receptionists for inclusion in appropriate general practice records. An example of a form in common use is shown in Figure 2.1. This form can be used to pass on details of out-of-hours visits made to patients of other practices being covered. There is a case for making notes of all telephone advice given, whether or not a visit is made.

```
┌─────────────────────────────────────────────────────────┐
│                      VISIT SLIP                           │
│                                                           │
│   NAME OF PATIENT: ....................................... │
│                                                           │
│   ADDRESS: ............................................... │
│                                                           │
│   DATE OF VISIT: ............. TIME OF VISIT: ............ │
│                                                           │
│   PRESENTING COMPLAINT: .................................. │
│                                                           │
│   ........................................................ │
│                                                           │
│   CLINICAL FINDINGS: ..................................... │
│                                                           │
│   ........................................................ │
│                                                           │
│   TREATMENT GIVEN: ....................................... │
│                                                           │
│   ........................................................ │
└─────────────────────────────────────────────────────────┘
```

Fig. 2.1. An example of a form commonly used to record details of out-of-hours visits.

References

1. Cole, F. H. (1981). The British Telecom radio-paging service in general practice. *J. Roy. Coll. Gen. Pract.*, **31**, 621–3.
2. Powell, H. (1987). Job sharing in practice. *GMSC Voice*, **4**, 14–15.
3. Sheldon, M. G. and Harris, S. J. (1984). Use of deputising services and night visit rates in general practice. *Brit. Med. J.*, **289**, 474–6.
4. Sawyer, L. and Arber, S. (1982). Changes in home visiting and night and weekend cover: the patient's view. *Brit. Med. J.*, **284**, 1531–4.
5. Riddell, J. A. (1980). Out-of-hours visits in a group practice. *Brit. Med. J.*, **280**, 1518–19.
6. Stevenson, J. S. K. (1982). Advantages of deputising services: a personal view. *Brit. Med. J.*, **284**, 947–9.
7. Tayside Area Health Board (1987). General Practice Subcommittee: Tayside Region. *Criteria for appointment as trainer.*
8. Skua. Deputising Diary (1987). *Scottish Medicine*, **5**, 15–16.

3 General principles

Patients' views

When someone is sufficiently ill to require medical attention outside normal surgery hours this generally implies more serious illness and greater anxiety, and for that reason people particularly want to see their own doctor, whom they know and trust, or a doctor from their own practice, who at least will not be totally unfamiliar.[1]

Such an ideal has to be seen against needs of doctors (and their families) to have appropriate leisure and recreation time. In 1984 almost two-thirds of a sample of 818 UK general practitioners worked over 60 hours a week (and nearly one-fifth worked more than 90 hours).[2]

An equitable solution, therefore, would aim both to provide cover 24 hours a day, 365 days a year for the whole needs of the individual patient, and to have due regard for the future of general practice and the lives of those attracted to this discipline. Some compromise is therefore necessary.

Moves to increase quality of care as well as morale and status in general practice have included a growing use of rota systems and deputizing services for out-of-hours cover.[3] Such off-duty arrangements have been the subject of criticism over the years, both in the UK and elsewhere in Northern Europe.[4] In general, however, off-duty arrangements appear to be acceptable to patients, though levels of public satisfaction with commercial deputizing services are considerably lower than with rota systems.[1]

How out-of-hours calls arise

Ways in which out-of-hours calls arise and are transmitted are usually much more complex than they appear. One indication of this is the fact that practices vary considerably in their night-visiting rates.[5] Even when they work from the same health centre, with no major demographic differences between the practices, and participate in the same organization for night-cover, different practices may have widely different night visiting rates—ranging in one recent study from 25.8 to 43.5 per thousand patients per year[6]—and the variation in rates of incoming telephone requests can be even higher. (Personal communication from J. A. R. Lawson, Dundee University Department of General Practice, 1988.) Such differences have not so far been fully explained, but expectations patients may have of their doctors, ways in which they may have been educated to use the services, and doctor–patient relationships probably all play a part.

The nature of the physical disease and its manifestations are important determinants, but demand is also conditioned by many other considerations, including how the patient perceives illness, the patient's and family's previous experiences of disease and of medical responses, together with all sorts of modifying factors, among which are featured patients' awareness of 'antisocial hours'.[7]

Although it may not always appear so to a general practitioner when he is on call, most people have a remarkably high threshold for 'bothering the family doctor': this features among reasons for out-of-hours self-referral to hospital accident and emergency departments[8]—as well as alegations about general practitioners' non-availability.

Contacting the doctor

Once the patient and/or relatives have decided to 'bother the doctor', a request for out-of-hours help is usually transmitted by telephone, more often than not through an intermediary.[9] It is from households without a telephone that out-of-hours calls are more likely to come;[10] these callers' problems of access may be compounded by the non-availability of public telephones, often as the result of vandalism.

Most callers do not experience major difficulties in contacting general practitioner services out ot hours,[11] but the process can be rather tortuous, involving more than two telephone calls, each stage adding its quota of exasperation to the mental condition of a caller who may already be anxious.

The author attempted to contact by telephone a sample of 25 separate practices (approximately one-third of Tayside's 300 principals in NHS general practice) out-of-hours at Christmas 1987. It did not prove possible to speak immediately to a pre-determined named doctor. All unengaged numbers were answered promptly (within 8 'rings') except in the case of one practice. Half of the practices contacted responded with a human voice, the remainder by answering machines. In about one-third, the messages had been recorded by the doctor: this can confuse the anxious patient (see p. 24). One practice using an answering machine also employed automatic transfer, so that the caller was put in contact with the duty doctor without having to dial a separate number. Contacts were made with a partner in the practice or a member of a small rota in over half the calls. In only two instances were the Tayside Deputizing Services involved.

Other parts of the country show some variations,[12] and Tayside doctors make less use of professional deputizing services than most other areas in the UK (a current estimate of the national scene suggests over 40 per cent of general practitioners use deputizing services).[13]

The Tayside study did not confirm an earlier impression that central telephone exchanges (intercept) are slow to answer: telephone operators were prompt to respond and articulate in their replies. Experience of the recorded messages in answering machines used in some practices was less reassuring. Some of the messages were given too quickly, and in at least one instance a further call was required to obtain the telephone number to which the caller was being re-directed.

Callers, needs, and demands

At the outset, it is as well to remember that, from the caller's point of view, 'trivial' and 'irresponsible' calls rarely, if ever, exist. Doctors vary in their views, and figures for this element vary from 86 per cent[14] down to zero.[15] Most reports suggest that the proportion of truly irresponsible or malicious calls is very small.

Some characteristics of callers

Using his background knowledge of the patients in his practice, supported by indirect measures of neuroticism, Jacob[16] concluded that late-callers in his practice were more prone to anxiety. One effect of the patient's age detected in his study was that a higher proportion of 'true' emergencies occurred among older patients. A relatively small proportion of the practice generated high demand, including out-of-hours calls.

Establishing identities and expectations

For reasons, some of which have already been discussed, out-of-hours calls share with most emergency calls a number of features, including a heightened emotional temperature (of the caller—and sometimes the doctor). Relevant factors include a perception by a lay person of the urgency of a situation as being of sufficient magnitude to 'bother the doctor'. The degree of urgency is usually assessed by the lay caller at a higher level than it is by the professional responder.[17] Much less frequently, however, the reverse is true: an anonymous article[18] in the series 'Mea Culpa' gives an in-depth narrative account of one such situation involving a persistently crying baby.

A second factor, encouraging a tendency to overstate the case, is the transmission of the message at second, third, or even fourth, hand. Opportunities for misunderstandings may also be compounded by 'the turn of the screw': here, at each relay, a slight but *deliberate* twist is given to the content, with the aim of ensuring that the doctor not only receives the message promptly, but gives it high priority. So, for example, a message which started as a request for advice about an irregular and unusually heavy menstrual period, may be transformed into 'Tell the doctor to come at once, she's *haemorrhaging*'.

Several points follow from this heightened emotional temperature. The caller, in the anxiety to get the message across, may launch straight into the account, and ring off without the necessary identities and addresses being established. It is therefore good practice for the *doctor* to establish *at the outset* the identity of the caller, the name of the patient, and where the patient is at the time; and it may be necessary firmly to interrupt the caller's message for this purpose. A more extreme example, linked with 'emotional deafness' sometimes associated with anxiety, is provided by the situation in which a telephone answering machine is involved. The anxious caller may mistake for a live conversation what is in fact a recorded message (especially if it has been recorded by the doctor, and his voice is known to the caller). For this reason, it is probably safer for the receptionist or some other party to provide the recorded message when an answering machine is used.

Sometimes the caller contacts the wrong doctor. This error may be quickly identified if the doctor knows the patients on the practice list; it becomes more difficult in a large group practice, and when the doctor is on call as part of a rota. It is always worthwhile establishing as far as possible on whose NHS list the patient's name is registered; but it is the patient's need which is of major importance in making a decision on whether or not to visit.

Who is your patient?

The current view in medical protection circles is clearly set out by Fulton (1988).[19] *The* consideration is the patient's need, and this overrides the question of whether or not the patient is on the practice list. For example, *When a visit is indicated*, under the NHS terms and conditions of service the doctor must attend and treat a temporary resident or an emergency at any address within the area of the practice, as set out in the local list of general practitioners, whether or not the doctor has a patient living at that address: a very good reason for limiting and delineating the area of the practice. If the doctor does not restrict the right to accept a patient (or keep an existing patient on the list at an address outside that area) a contract is created, perhaps even by use and wont, to visit at that address at any time the need arises.

The 'emotional temperature'

It is also worthwhile attempting to gauge the 'emotional temperature' at this stage. If this is not done, the possibility exists for 'crossing the lines', in terms of transactional analysis,[20] and responding inappropriately on what the doctor may mistakenly believe to be an adult-to-adult level. The risk here is that the caller becomes angry and 'hangs up' prematurely, so that the whole call for help may be frustrated.

As in all medical communications, the replacement of emotionally neutral words (such as 'faint') by emotionally charged terms (such as 'collapse'), combined with a rapid delivery and a raised tone of voice, is a hallmark of anxiety.

Example 1 (transcription of a 2 a.m. call to a sudden death)

Caller: Mr . . . speaking. Something queer is happening to my wife.
I-I-I don't know. She seems to be collapsed completely in
bed, you know. Terrific pain under the left-hand side. I've
tried to give her a cup of tea, but I think she's away.

(The patient had in fact sustained a rapidly fatal myocardial
infarct.)

Another lead into emotional assessment is given by the
presence or absence of internal consistency in the message.
If the caller describes actions by the patient that are incon-
sistent with the supposed health problem, or if, in repeating
the main facts, the caller paints a different picture from that
originally projected, one reason might be anxiety.

Prior knowledge can play a major role in a decision to
visit;[21] information concerning the patient and the household
from which the call originates is often available to the family
doctor. This knowledge may allow the doctor to make appropriate adjustments in his professional assessment of need as
opposed to reacting to the urgency of lay demand.

Example 2

The 10 p.m. caller sought help for her mother, who had
developed swelling of the leg.

In this instance the doctor had the following prior knowledge:

1. The patient (caller's mother) was a responsible person.
2. The daughter (the caller) was a staff nurse.
3. The patient's husband was in hospital with inoperable
   lung cancer.

Because of knowledge such as this, the family doctor may
respond to apparently similar requests in widely differing
ways which, to the external observer, might appear to be
idiosyncratic. This aspect of telephone calls, of value in telephone decision-making at the level of the individual patient,

is usually the result of years of experience of the people concerned, and so is denied the trainee or new entrant to general practice. If the doctor interposes an intermediary (for example, a caretaker living over the surgery premises) who has to relay calls, some of the doctor's personal knowledge cannot be applied. Most calls in these circumstances are thereby more likely to be converted into visits.

Deciphering the message

Callers often do not express clearly what they expect of the doctor. It is therefore important for the doctor consciously to aim at a diagnosis or formulation of the problems of the 'intermediary', to help him (or her) with his needs and anxieties.[22] Sometimes, as in the transcript of the 2 a.m. call (p. 26), the starkness of the message crystallizes the situation (and its implications for the doctor). More frequently the situation is less clear.

Example 3

9 p.m. Caller: I'm actually on a switchboard, but my son-in-law has just come on this phone to me. (Dr: 'Yes'.) Baby's due on 29 January. (Dr: 'Uh huh'.) It's Pamela, my daughter: she's had this pain, as though it was a nerve, you know ... (Dr: 'Mm mm'.) since before 3 o'clock today (Dr: 'Mm mm'.) and it's still there. And the last time she had to get the inspection for her dates (Dr: 'Yes'.) and seemingly the head wasn't engaged or something. I mean I am rather worried too (Dr: 'Yes'.) and I just don't know what to do. You see, he came on to ask me; you see; they're young. (Dr: 'Mm mm'.) And I says, "Well, if you'll hold on the line, I'll phone and ask the doctor what to do ...".

In the transcript above, the caller does not firmly request a visit, and the doctor may legitimately wonder who exactly is the patient. Sometimes, however, even if no firm request is made for a visit, and in the absence of a stark message, some clinical problems will point to the need to supplement the telephoned information with an early objective examination: some of the more obvious examples include:

- trauma;
- sudden onset of chest pain (especially in middle-aged men);
- the persistently crying child;
- abdominal pain in children;
- sudden severe shortness of breath;
- loss of consciousness and slow recovery;
- severe pain; and
- blood loss.

Doctors and the telephone

Before considering in greater detail the nature and range of options available for out-of-hours clinical decison-making, effects on the doctor of providing cover are discussed, because merely being on-call can be stressful to the doctor (and his family), whether or not patients actually call on the general practitioner's services.

Stress and emotion

Samuel[23] describes what he calls 'paranoid telephone tinnitus", in which any ringing sound produces an alarm reaction in the doctor; and, although his article is written in a humorous vein, many general practitioners will immediately recognize this state. Hospital doctors, too, may feel stressed by the telephone; but the general practitioner has the added 'surprise element', in that his out-of-hours calls have not first been processed by a professional (whether nurse or junior doctor).

Another, and obvious, stress factor is the disruption of

sleep. It appears that interruption may be as disruptive as actual loss of sleep; especially a telephone call during the first hour of sleep, whether a home visit is made or not.

A nagging feeling expressed by some that the history elicited via the telephone through a third party is always insufficient for rational management decisions may not accord with the facts; but the feeling is real enough, and adds its contribution to the stress doctors experience. Sometimes this is compounded by other emotions, prominent among which, in many caring doctors, is a sense of guilt when the doctor contrives to turn an ill-expressed request for a visit into a telephone-advice interaction: together with the observation that many young and/or single parents are ill-equipped to cope, even with advice, this is a factor which contributes to the relatively high night-visiting rates in areas of multiple deprivation.[24]

Anger is another emotion, more usually evident in the caller than in the doctor. Reasons why the caller's emotional temperature may be raised have already been discussed: its importance is its potential for disrupting communication before the relevant information has been imparted to the doctor. Some of the heat may quickly be taken out of the situation by the doctor making clear at the outset that he is very willing to visit: occasionally, and in suitable circumstances, this move can turn a caller's preremptory order to visit into a more rational advice-giving exchange, even ending with the caller apologizing for any rudeness!

For these and other reasons, a case may be made for ensuring for the doctor adequate time off following on-call duties,[25] though few practices appear to build this into their organization.

Options and responses

At the outset, it should be stated that the response a doctor makes, whether or not to visit, for example, is his professional responsibility. Under the terms and conditions of service in the National Health Service a general practitioner is *not* obliged to respond with a visit, even if such a request is explicitly made by the caller. If, however, the patient comes to harm, and it can be shown to relate to the doctor's failure to visit, the doctor may face an action for damages and/or reprimand by the NHS.

Several options are open to the doctor in making decisions on management. They include:

- home visit;
- telephone advice—how to cope within the family
                  —to come to the surgery
                  —to go to the local Accident and
                    Emergency Department;
- admit to hospital (without visiting); and
- other.

To visit?

A decision to visit is often best for the patient and prudent for the doctor, because it affords the doctor the objective evidence he will otherwise lack.

In addition, it will often allow him to cope more fully with the 'intermediary' (who may have initiated the call), relatives, and 'significant others' when their disturbed state is much greater than that of the patient, as is sometimes the case. Furthermore, it meets expectations society has of general practitioners in the UK.

The decision may be determined by the nature of the physical problems, such as those listed on p. 28.

A high degree of anxiety is commonly present in the attendants, but some other situations in themselves are of such emotional intensity as to warrant prompt visiting: they include bereavement (especially the loss of a child) and major depressive illness. Social determinants too may operate: for example, the doctor's appreciation of the wish of the caller to share responsibility (for instance, wardens of sheltered housing, or the caring staff of residential homes for the elderly). The social isolation of the patient, and the burdens of loneliness, may exert lesser pressures. The doctor's awareness of a background of possible social deprivation is another factor in deciding to visit[24] rather than give advice.

Other determinants in an otherwise 'doubtful' request include factors such as the doctor's commitment, already made separately, to visit another patient in the neighbourhood of the call.

A second unsolicited request from a caller whose previous call has been managed by 'advice only' should result in a visit, whether or not this has been clearly requested by the caller. Another general principle is 'when in doubt, visit'.

When to visit?

Once a decision to visit has been made, the doctor has still to order its priority. Should it be done immediately? One suggested scheme[26] for categorizing urgency is as follows:

High: urgent treatment necessary to avoid severe suffering or risk of serious deterioration (visits after a patient's death included);

Medium: symptoms or circumstances sufficiently concerning to justify an out-of-hours visit, where prompt treatment would facilitate recovery;

Low: minor illness or discomfort not justifying an out-of-hours visit; delay in diagnosis or treatment would not lengthen the recovery period; other patients with the same complaint would have managed it themselves.

In one study of 296 home visits, to which the above classification was applied retrospectively, 41 per cent were judged as high, 3 per cent medium, and 17 per cent low. However, selectivity in deciding to make a visit was higher than that evident in other reported studies, and the proportion of telephone advice was correspondingly high (58.6 per cent). Clinical circumstances are a key determinant here. Most general practitioners would wish to attend major medical (in the wide sense) emergencies as soon as possible. There are, however, a number of other considerations which may influence the timing of the visit when urgency is professionally assessed at a lower level. The anxious parent (whose child is heard howling lustily in the background) may be perpetuating her child's discomfort by her own anxiety: once this is relieved—and merely contacting the doctor may have this effect—calm may be restored. It is worth while allowing sufficient time for this to happen, and the visit can then concentrate on building up the parent's confidence. The doctor may also wish to delay visiting until a number of calls are accumulated, possibly thereby increasing efficiency in providing this resource.

On the other hand, the rapidity with which the doctor responds to a request with a visit has been identified as an important element in promoting a high degree of patient satisfaction—second only to 'which doctor it was who made the call'.[27]

Where to visit?

The importance of establishing the *location* of the patient was stressed on p. 24. This is not synonymous with 'address', because in emergencies patients, especially if living alone, may move their abode.

It is always worth asking the caller for specific instructions on how to find the house when there is any doubt. Most general practitioners have experienced the sometimes grossly inadequate means of street identification, and the mad logic of house numbering—confusion worse confounded by darkness, non-existent street lighting, inclement weather, and the effects of vandalism! In such circumstances, it helps if the house to be visited can be appropriately lit up, and the caller should be asked to take suitable action.

Meeting at the surgery

Sometimes, when the doctor judges it desirable to see the patient, instead of visiting the patient's home, he may ask the caller to bring the patient to the surgery or to his house out-of-hours. (The use of the doctor's house in this way varies among practices, and is perhaps commoner in rural and semi-rural areas. See Appendix 2.) Such a request would, of course, be contingent on suitable transport being available for the patient. Such advice would be appropriate for Saturday afternoon and Sunday calls, for injured patients who may be better dealt with in the treatment room, and situations where the patient's notes may need to be consulted or where medication not in the doctor's bag may be needed. There may be psychological merit in relatives (and patients) having to make some investment in the management of their problems.

Not to visit

Rarely a decision has to be firmly made *not* to become involved. Situations in which drunken behaviour and violence feature may be handled more appropriately by the police. A recent and unpleasant development is the deliberate manipulation of the doctor by drug abusers intent on obtaining dangerous drugs. Such a call may not always be readily identified, because some drug abusers have become skilled in putting across spurious messages, prominent among which is 'bleeding'. If the doctor is in any doubt on this score, he should decide either not to visit (and record in the medical case notes his decision together with the reasons for it), or to make a visit with a police escort.

Domestic violence is another situation where the family doctor might properly refuse to become involved; but if he does, he should be very wary about appearing to take sides in family squabbles.

Occasionally a request received shortly before 'handing back' may appropriately be left to a doctor with whom the patient is more familiar. The early-rising (and sometimes confused) elderly patient, whose condition does not appear to be urgent, is one such example.

Efficient care and patient education

If it is accepted that only about a half of requests for out-of-hours help require the services of a doctor,[28] and that not all calls represent emergencies, a visit in response to every call would not only be inefficient, but might preclude a prompt response to calls of greater urgency. In addition, too ready a willingness to visit, coupled with an uncritical kind of decision-making, might result in encouraging some households to expect inappropriate visiting, and in the creation of undesirable doctor-dependency.[29] These and other arguments have been adduced in the debate on whether or not general practitioners in the UK should increase their use of telephone advice.[26]

Consultations in general practice afford opportunities for doctors to educate patients and their families to make better or more appropriate use of medical services.[30] A need to stress this aspect of care is often apparent during out-of-hours visits; it may be that a family could have been managed appropriately without a visit, or that when faced with the same situation next time a family could take action which would obviate the need for the doctor's presence. Care needs to be exercised in how and when this education is achieved, in order to avoid giving unnecessary offence. The subject is best broached once the presenting situation has been dealt with, and the emotional temperature has been lowered.

Giving advice over the telephone

A considerable proportion (between one- and two-thirds) of requests may be met appropriately with advice. Elements in this management decision are:

- providing a listening ear;
- finding out what has already been done;
- ensuring the caller understands what is involved; and
- leaving specific instructions to call again later the same evening if still troubled.

Some form of more definitive follow-up is indicated in a proportion of such calls: this may help to prevent the episode which occasioned the out-of-hours call from drifting into a state of indeterminate illness. The caller (or patient) should then be invited to make a follow-up appointment—or a visit later in the week may be agreed upon.

Among other elements in good telephone management Marsh et al.[26] identify the following:

- The ideal that the doctor himself should whenever possible speak to the patient.
- The importance of the personal link between doctor and patient in promoting confidence.
- Appointments readily available as soon as the surgery opens.
- Knowing from the address and other data whether the patient is living in deprived circumstances.
- A welcoming attitude to the caller on the part of the doctor.
- Instructions to ring back if the problem persists.

It is suggested that other practices, by applying such criteria, might increase their efficiency without detriment to patient care, though this is hotly disputed by some.[31]

A small number of patients (among them some single parents) are characterized by 'acting on a short fuse'. If a demand for a visit is not met immediately, such patients or their associates may put pressure on the general practitioner by threatening him in a variety of ways—reporting him to 'the Authorities' or, more subtly, by stating an intention to go straight to hospital. If the threats are resisted, it is sometimes worth while alerting the ambulance controller or the appropriate hospital about the possibility of inappropriate calls being made on those services.

Direct referral

Sometimes the doctor's response to an emergency call will be advice to take the patient direct to hospital without the customary visit. Such action does not always strengthen relationships between general practitioners and hospitals, but it may be called for in special circumstances. Examples include a severe medical condition combined with the patient's closer proximity to the hospital, the on-call doctor having to deal simultaneously with two (or rarely more) major emergencies when other members of the rota are unavailable, or the doctor's becoming immobilized (for instance, in a heavy snowfall). Inter-professional relationships may be preserved by a phone call beforehand to the hospital concerned, explaining the special circumstances.

Mobilizing other help

Quite apart from the general consideration that approximately one half of out-of-hours calls should be managed by a nurse,[28] there are occasions when the problem, after prior filtering by the doctor, can properly be delegated to other members of the primary care team. It might be appropriate, for example, for the doctor to relay directly to the nurse a request from a patient with a blocked in-dwelling catheter, or the distressed elderly with faecal impaction. Willingness to become so involved on the part of other members of the primary care team could improve the quality of care. For example, a Health Visitor who makes available her home telephone number for out-of-hours consultations can spare the doctor, and ensure for her clients a possibly more suitable source of sound advice.

Experience of the work of a night duty health visitor service in North London[32] showed that it could usefully supplement general practitioner services (especially in an area where deputizing services are operated).

The 'heavy breathing call'

Most general practitioners and their households are familiar with the telephone call which, as soon as it is answered, is abruptly terminted by the caller without a word, and sometimes after a short period of heavy breathing. The significance of such calls (which may constitute less than one per cent) cannot easily be determined—some may simply be the result of misdialling, others the work of mischief; but some are likely to be the effect on a caller of failing to make direct contact with the personal doctor he or she wishes to contact. Doctors' families should be prepared not to be disturbed by such calls.

References

1. Sawyer, L. and Arber, S. (1982). Changes in home visiting and night and weekend cover: the patient's view. *Brit. Med. J.*, **284**, 1531–4.
2. Anonymous (1984). Survey of GP's attitudes to out-of-hours cover. *Brit. Med. J.*, **288**, 1627.

3. Roland, M. (1984). Deputising services. *Brit. Med. J.*, **289**, 451–2.
4. Hall, D. W. (1975). The off-duty arrangements of general practitioners in four European countries. *J. Roy. Coll. Gen. Pract.*, **26**, 19–34.
5. Sheldon, M. G. and Harris, S. J. (1984). Use of deputising services and night visit rates in general practice. *Brit. Med. J.*, **289**, 474–6.
6. Usherwood, T. P., Kapasi, M. A., and Barber, J. H. (1985). Wide variations in night visiting rate. *J. Roy. Coll. Gen. Pract.*, **35**, 395.
7. Campion, P. D. and Gabriel, J. (1985). Illness behaviour in mothers with young chldren. *Soc. Sci. Med.*, **20**, 325–30.
8. Calnan, M. (1983). Managing 'minor' disorders: pathways to a hospital accident and emergency department. *Sociology of Health and Illness*, **5**, 149–7.
9. Bailey, A. J. (1979). Home visiting: the part played by the "intermediary". *J. Roy. Coll. Gen. Pract.*, **29**, 137–42.
10. Riddell, J. A. (1980). Out-of-hours visits in a group practice. *Brit. Med. J.*, **280**, 1518–19.
11. Ritchie, J., Jacoby, A., and Bone, M. (1981). *Access to primary health care*, Office of Population Censuses and Surveys. HMSO, London.
12. Lyall, J. (1978). The call of duty. *General Practitioner* 24 March.
13. Martin, P., Moulds, A. J., and Kerrigan, P. J. C. (1985). In *Towards better practice*, Library of General Practice, p. 70. Churchill Livingstone, London.
14. Gabriel, R. (1976). Emergency call service. *J. Roy. Coll. Gen. Pract.*, **26**, 74–5.
15. Barley, S. L. (1979). Night calls in group practice. *J. Roy. Coll. Gen. Pract.*, **29**, 752–3.
16. Jacob, A. (1963). The personal characteristics of people who require late calls. *J. Roy. Coll. Gen. Pract.*, **6**, 436–47.
17. Barber, J. H., Moore, M. F., Robinson, E. T., and Taylor, T. R. (1976). Urgency and risk in first contact decisions in general practice. *Health Bulletin*, **34**, 21–9.
18. Anonymous (1987). *Mea culpa*: failure to visit a crying baby. *Update*, **35**, 1242.
19. Fulton, W. W. (1988). Terms of service for doctors. In *Annual Report 1988*, p. 14. The Medical and Dental Defence Union of Scotland.

20. Berne, E. (1964). *Games people play.* Penguin Books, London.
21. Crowe, M. G. F., Hurwood, D. S., and Taylor, R. W. (1976). Out-of-hours calls in a Leicestershire practice. *Brit. Med. J.*, **1**, 1582–4.
22. Bailey, A. J. (1979). Home visiting: the part played by the "intermediary". *J. Roy. Coll. Gen. Pract.*, **29**, 137–42.
23. Samuel, O. (1983). What annoys me most: the telephone. *Brit. Med. J.*, **287**, 1599–1600.
24. Riddell, J. A. (1980). Out-of-hours visits in a group practice. *Brit. Med. J.*, **280**, 1518–19.
25. Pitts, J. (1988). Hours of work and fatigue in doctors. *J. Roy. Coll. Gen. Pract.*, **38**, 2–3.
26. Marsh, G. N., Horne, R. A., and Channing, D. M. (1987). A study of telephone advice in managing out-of-hours calls. *J. Roy. Coll. Gen. Pract.*, **37**, 301–4.
27. Sawyer, L. and Arber, S. (1982). Changes in home visiting and night and weekend cover: the patient's view. *Brit. Med. J.*, **284**, 1531–4.
28. Tulloch, A. J. (1984). Out-of-hours calls in an Oxfordshire practice. *Practitioner*, **228**, 663–8.
29. Cubitt, T. and Tobias, G. (1983). Out of hours calls in general practice: does the doctor's attitude alter patient demands? *Brit. Med. J.*, **287**, 28–30.
30. Stott, N. C. H. (1983). *Primary health care.* Springer-Verlag, Berlin.
31. Berrow, P. J. (1987). Telephone advice in managing out-of-hours calls. *J. Roy. Coll. Gen. Pract.*, **37**, 463.
32. Littlewood, J. (1986). Out-of-hours calls revisited. *J. Roy. Coll. Gen. Pract.*, **36**, 85.

4 Tactics

For most doctors, the most usual response to an out-of-hours telephone call will be to make a visit. Out-of-hours house calls, like out-of-hours phone calls, are a little different from home visiting during the day.

Some features of visits

The visit may be to a patient of another practice, and the circumstances and address may be unfamiliar. The medical records may not be available, and even if they are, the complex security systems of some surgery premises may act as a disincentive to the doctor wishing to gain access to them.[1] Darkness, lack of adequate street lighting, and vandalism may add to difficulties in locating the patient. In areas of urban deprivation, possibilities of physical violence to the doctor exist,[2] especially at night. The request may be made to appear more urgent so that the doctor is more likely to carry with him the emergency bag, with its supplies of abusable drugs. Because he may be the only doctor on call, back-up from other doctors, normally present during the day, may be less readily available, and, of course, he must make special arrangements to ensure that the telephone is manned in his absence. Traffic is usually less, and travelling times are shorter: the sporadic nature of out-of-hours calls also reduces the opportunities for the economic route-planning necessary for groups of visits during the day. When the house-call is actually paid, the patient's household, because of a lack of preparation for the doctor's visit, sometimes gives a much clearer impression of how its members live; and often there are more people present than is the case during the day. The clinical problems have a different set of probabilities. Obtaining medication from the retail pharmacist is an option not so readily open to relatives, and in treating the condition the doctor is more likely to administer the medication directly than to give a drug by prescription. In making follow-up arrangements the doctor may have to consider his colleague's ways of practice, which he would not normally have to do with his own patients visited during the day.

Some of these factors are discussed more fully because of the implications they may have for the speedy and effective delivery of out-of-hours care.

Selective preparedness

Because of the recent increase in cases of the doctor's car being broken into and dangerous drugs being stolen, some general practitioners no longer carry their emergency bags. In dealing with out-of-hours requests it is important for the doctor to have information on which to base decisions on *both* the urgency *and* the probable nature of health problems. He will then decide whether or not to take the emergency bag (which personal experience suggests is required in less than one in twenty visits made), and/or special additional equipment such as a portable nebulizer and/or electrocardiograph. This is an area of decision-making where prior knowledge of the patient is extremely useful. Where this is not available first-hand, it may be worth while making a detour to the surgery to consult the medical record, even though this may add to the interval between telephone call and house call. It is good practice for colleagues working in a rota to alert the doctor on-call to the possibility that patients with problems may put in a call during the off-duty period, and to give background information.

Patients and some common problems

In a publication such as this it would be inappropriate to discuss clinical diagnosis and management of medical emergencies in detail: other works deal exhaustively with these subjects. There are, however, a number of matters of a more general nature which it is useful to keep in mind when dealing with some groups of conditions. Here are a few examples:

New babies

Most young parents probably experience their greatest insecurity in dealing with neonatal physiological phenomena such as crying, 'possetting' (regurgitating curdled milk), and transient skin manifestation. Their judgement on when to call for help is often exercised for the first time. It is easy for the insensitive doctor to destroy confidence by well-intentioned actions: for example by picking up and successfully soothing a healthy, angry baby. Heavy-handed attempts to minimize the seriousness of a situation in an effort to allay anxiety can lead to a loss of 'face'. By the same token, these contacts provide special opportunities for educating parents in the appropriate use of general practitioner services, an integral part of many a consultation whenever it occurs.[3]

Young babies

Parents' anxieties are again prominent, as exemplified by the common though ill-understood 'evening colic'[4] of the two to four month old baby. It is well for the doctor to remember that the parents' awareness of catastrophes such as sudden infant death or meningitis may already be heightened by the mass media. Such heightened anxieties can contribute to a child's distress whatever the diagnosis, and allaying parents' fears is as important as dealing with the baby's condition.

Older children

The evening rise in temperature in a pyrexial patient has been mentioned. There exists a medical view[5] that, provided the temperature rise does not constitute hyperpyrexia, such a positive and helpful part of the body's reaction to infection should not be too energetically treated with antipyretics. Abdominal pain in children is usually associated with parental fear, often unexpressed, of a possible acute appendicitis. Such fears are usually groundless, and whenever the doctor senses their presence the subject should be broached.

Earache is another relatively common reason for out-of-hours visits. Should all cases be immediately treated by antibiotics? Such a management decision rests on insecure evidence;[6] but parental pressures may be hard to resist. The whole question of blind antibiotic therapy in the febrile child in general practice is hedged by uncertainties. Some pharmaceutical firms appear to be eager to exploit this situation by providing starter packs of antibiotics for the doctor's bag free of charge. However, one study provides no support for routine oral amoxycillin in febrile children with no focal bacterial disease.[7]

Night cough in children is not fully understood; but an aetiological factor may be a drop in the air temperature of the bedroom during the night. Management should therefore incorporate advice about appropriate background heating and humidity, especially in the case of laryngitis stridulosa ('croup').

Adults

Chest pain at night, especially in those known to suffer from angina, deserves special mention, because its mechanisms are not fully understood. In a rota with different doctors each night, it becomes all too easy for such a patient (and relatives) to be educated into expecting an immediate, though unnecessary, injection of some powerful analgesic, or admission to hospital for every twinge.

The *parenteral* administration of a drug to a patient at night can be a potent way of indicating to some families that not only has their out-of-hours call been justified, but also the patient is 'seriously' ill. If the patient happens to be a member of another practice, it becomes even more important to let the doctor know that a drug has been given *by injection* when 'handing over'.

The elderly

Exacerbation of confusion in the elderly at night may be minimized by ensuring the presence of a night-light, and securing for the patient appropriate companionship. Psychotropic therapy in this situation can exacerbate the problem, and its use calls for special clinical judgement.

A not uncommon out-of-hours call (at least in Scotland) to the elderly is that occasioned by 'collapse' in a church. Such a telephone call usually comes in around lunch-time. The clinical problem is often a cross between postural hypotension and a vasovagal attack, but the differential diagnosis is wide.

Relatives

The importance of the intermediary in out-of-hours telephone calls has been stressed (p. 21). Their role in the out-of-hours visit is equally important. Usually their anxiety level is high, and this situation may be handled by giving them something to do.

A phenomenon well known to most general practitioners is the week-end call from a friend or relative who appears on the scene for the first time during an episode of illness. Unaware of all that has been accomplished to ensure that the care of the patient (usually elderly) is continued in the community, and anxious to demonstrate concern for the patient, such a visitor sometimes initiates a Sunday call. This type of situation intensifies just before Christmas, and the doctor may feel he is being used almost like a Christmas card! Handling such situations calls for considerable diplomacy, because the origins of the call may lie in the guilt some relatives feel (especially when they live at a distance).

Week-end calls and visits

In addition to 'Sunday syncope' and 'the guilty relative syndrome', there are a number of other factors encountered on weekend out-of-hours calls. Sometimes a relative (often a child) is taken ill when visiting. The illness may be minor and, of itself, insufficient to call for medical help. Questions of fitness to travel and risks of infecting others when public transport is involved are then the matters about which advice is sought rather than treatment.

Some households lurch from crisis to crisis in ordinary living, and a call occasioned by the patient's merely running out of long-term medication is understandable: such a request in better educated or endowed households can sorely try the patience of even the most phlegmatic doctor!

Special availability

While all general practitioners, like others, are entitled to leisure time, and to having that leisure time respected, most are prepared to make themselves personally available, whether on-call or not, in some circumstances. This personal availability is of special importance in the management of the terminally ill at home.

Those general practitioners who continue to conduct intra-natal obstetrics may also feel the paramount importance of this personal relationship, continuing care as opposed to continuity of care.

The ready availability of personal family doctoring through the NHS has been in the past one reason for the relatively low proportion of 'truly private' patients in general practice: under a market-orientated policy this may change.

Patients in all the categories mentioned above may have special access to their family doctor—or be encouraged to contact him at his home telephone number.

Some general practitioners take a very firm line on protecting their households from intrusion, to the extent of publishing only the telephone number of their workplace, their home number being ex-directory. Such a move is understandable in certain areas where respect for persons, personal property, and a person's right to privacy is generally low. It may be perceived as an additional barrier by some patients, but perhaps more importantly it can interfere with communications between colleagues. Some Local Medical Committees circulate among their members a list of their ex-directory numbers.

Death and out-of-hours visits

Over and above all the usual implications deaths at home carry for the general practitioner, with regard to dealing with this situation out-of-hours a number of questions may be raised.

For example, is it necessary to visit immediately? The doctor's response to a death during the night, occurring in a nursing home, where it has been anticipated, may be different from the sudden death at home. In addition to comforting the bereaved it is a kindness to relatives (and of practical help to the undertaker) if the doctor lays out the body—occasionally a difficult task if the deceased is heavy, lying in a grotesque position, and contaminated with vomit, faeces, or blood. Relatives may need to be guided in delaying contacting the undertaker until next morning.

References

1. Riddell, J. A. (1980). Out-of-hours visits in a group practice. *Brit. Med. J.*, **280**, 1518–19.
2. Savage, R. (1984). Violence. *Brit. Med. J.*, **289**, 1518.
3. Stott, N. C. H. (1983). *Primary health care.* Springer-Verlag, Berlin.
4. Illingworth, R. S. (1952). Evening colic in infants. *Lancet*, **ii**, 1019–20.
5. Watson, G. I. (1982). In *Epidemiology and research in a general practice*, p. 77. Royal College of General Practitioners, London.
6. Jones, R. and Bain, J. (1986). Three-day and seven-day treatment in acute otitis media: a double-blind antibiotic trial. *J. Roy. Coll. Gen. Pract.*, **36**, 356–8.
7. Journal of the Royal College of General Practitioners (1988). Digest: antibiotics for the febrile child. *J. Roy. Coll. Gen. Pract.*, **38**, 38.

Envoi

The aim of this book is to provide the trainee general practitioner and other readers with a review of information culled from a range of different sources and interpreted in the light of the needs of both patients and family doctors. Political and fiscal aspects of out-of-hours work, important though they are, have received relatively little consideration: yet, if general practice is to continue to adapt to meet a changing situation, such considerations will become paramount.

Those who subscribe to the Leeuwenhorst definition[1] of the general practitioner, with its emphasis on personal, primary, and continuing care, will have no difficulty in accepting out-of-hours work as an essential constituent of the work of the family doctor. In its turn, a society which values its general practitioners will respect their right to leisure and privacy. The conflict inherent in these two concepts is heightened by a lack of understanding sometimes evident among patients on how out-of-hours services actually operate. A doctor's understandable desire to protect himself and his household from unwarranted invasion of privacy may have been heightened by a lack of purposeful training in telephone techniques and by rising expectations of the Welfare State. Means of resolving the problems are being afforded by technological developments, but these may also be perceived by patients to be barriers to communication. It seems appropriate therefore that the public's use of out-of-hours general practitioner services should be a legitimate subject to include in health education in general. At the level of the practice, whatever system operates, the patients should be briefed as fully as the circumstances indicate: if out of hours they are usually required to make two or more calls before making contact with the doctor, and if a deputizing service is regularly used, then they may feel entitled to know this.

The doctor's handling of telephone requests is largely, though not entirely, a matter of common sense. There is room for relevant contributions to both undergraduate education and postgraduate training, with the proviso that the diverse circumstances of general practice be taken fully into account.

There appears to be a place for greater experiment in ways in which out-of-hours calls are handled. If a relatively high proportion of calls do not need to be responded to in purely 'medical' terms, and if there is scope for extending telephone advice, then a logical development might be to apply a primary-care team approach: health visitor, nursing sister, and doctor might *all* share in out-of-hours practice work to the benefit of the patient, taking turns to be 'on call', and prepared to delegate as might be indicated.

Few general practitioners would cavil at the suggestion that much more must be done by local authorities to help emergency services to locate those in need of these services, especially at night.

It is difficult to reconcile the aims of the general practitioner who seeks more leisure time with those of colleagues willing to continue to provide a 24-hours service, but who feel that, under current NHS regulations, the rewards for this are derisory.

The 1988 annual report of the General Medical Services Committee contains a succinct section on out-of-hours work. The case for re-negotiation of terms of service to a more work-sensitive contract is reviewed, and seven options are briefly discussed.

These options consist of:

- higher remuneration without detriment to normal-hours remuneration;
- re-distribution from normal hours to out-of-hours;

- a right to opt out of out-of-hours work;
- payment by the patient;
- extension of hours which attract item-of-service payments;
- higher fees for doctors who attend personally; and
- unrestricted freedom to use deputizing services.

It is not the author's intention unfairly to criticize the use of deputizing services. However, if society shares the author's belief in the value of a personalized medical service, in the need to struggle to secure such care and maintain it at an appropriately high standard, then it must find the necessary resources and the political will for this to happen. Without it, general practice and our patients will be the poorer.

References

1. European Conference on the Teaching of General Practice (1977). The work of the general practitioner—Leeuwenhorst Working Party Report. *J. Roy. Coll. Gen. Pract.*; **27**, 117.

Appendix 1: A code of out-of-hours telephone practice

The following section draws heavily on the report of the Working Group appointed by the General Medical Services Committee to study telephone answering services; it also takes account of the published work cited in the bibliography. The author, however, accepts full responsibility for the views expressed.

1. It is the general practitioner's responsibility to make adequate arrangements for receiving and transmitting messages out-of-hours.

2. The general practitioner should ensure that the information in the NHS Medical List and in the telephone directory is up-to-date—and is kept up-to-date.

3. The practice should ensure that patients are adequately informed about how the practice operates out-of-hours. Such information should be considered for inclusion in the practice brochure—if one is available.

4. The practice might review annually its policy on out-of-hours calls—the review preferably to be based on the sort of data illustrated in Appendix 2. The review should consider the following details:

   • out-of-hours contact with a *doctor* should normally be feasible by calling not more than two different numbers, and after a total of two attempts;

   • where possible, the caller makes contact by the second attempt, and informed *dialogue* is possible between caller and recipient; and

- where taped messages are used, they should be of good quality, easily understood, with clear instructions, preferably recorded by someone other than the doctor, and repeated at least once.

5. Where deputizing services are used, from time to time a practice should attempt to find out whether the arrangements suit its patients. It should consider critically whether the professional decisions these services make about their patients are of a standard at least comparable to that which the practice doctor would regard as appropriate. The practice could review at least annually the use made of commercial deputizing services: in the case of a group practice making regular use of such services, the situation might be re-appraised with a view to a possible reduction of such usage, replacing it with a rota where possible.

6. In dealing with callers, the doctor should take account of the problems of the intermediary as well as of the patient, and at the outset of the conversation should make clear a willingness to visit where this seems appropriate.

7. Identification and location of the patient should also be established early on during the telephone call.

8. When the doctor gives advice he should ensure that it is properly understood, getting the caller to repeat it if necessary. The caller should be asked to phone back if the problem does not seem to be easing.

9. The doctor should ensure that the phone-sitter can contact him (by radio-pager or other means) when he leaves home to make a visit.

10. When in doubt—visit.

Appendix 2: An audit of out-of-hours calls

An audit of out-of-hours calls in a semi-rural practice (9312 patients, five partners, and one trainee)

1987	Visits	Night visits 11p.m.-7a.m. (NV)	Advice	Night advice 11p.m.-7a.m. (NA)	Home* consult.	Messages	Night disturbance rate (NV + NA)	Total patient contact
Jan.	76	9	63	(8)	19	4	(17)	170
Feb.	81	11	64	(8)	13	—	(19)	169
March	74	16	57	(8)	15	—	(24)	162
April	55	7	44	(7)	17	5	(14)	128
May	61	11	36	—	17	3	(11)	128
June	56	14	41	(6)	16	3	(20)	130
July	46	9	50	(6)	14	2	(15)	121
August	47	7	44	(2)	11	—	(9)	109
Sept.	55	13	54	(8)	11	—	(21)	133
Oct.	65	3	52	(6)	9	3	(9)	132
Nov.	63	13	46	(8)	12	6	(21)	140
Dec.	74	8	60	(8)	24	8	(16)	176
Total	753	121	610	(75)	178	34	(196)	1696

*Home here means doctor's house.

By kind permission of Doctors Hepworth, D. M., McGill, J. S., Mackintosh, K. D., Macleod, H. D., and Russell, W. G., *Newport on Tay.*

These statistics can be compared with other practices as follows:

	Ourselves	Hobday	Gadsby	Marsh
Night visit rate/1000/annum	13.0	6.0	14.0	9.8
Night advice rate/1000/annum	8.0	10.2	6.0	13.6
Night disturbance rate	21.0	16.2	20.0	23.4
Out of hours				
Visit rate/1000 patients/annum	93.8	35.9	86.0	47.5
Phone calls/1000 patients/annum	69.1	102.4	84.0	76.1
Disturbance/1000 patients/annum	182.3	138.4	170.0	53.3
Per cent of calls managed by phone	37.0	74.0	49.0	58.6
Per cent requiring visits	63.0	26.0	51.0	36.6

Apart from statistical analysis the 'out-of-hours' diary has removed an area of laxity from our record keeping—the receptionists are recording each patient contact, with its content, in the patient records. It also ensures that none of our night visit fees are missed!

References

Gadsby, R. (1987). Telephone advice in managing out-of-hours calls. *J. Roy. Coll. Gen. Pract.*, **37**, 462.

Hobday, P. J. (1984). Night workload in one health district. *Brit. Med. J.*, **289**, 663–4.

Marsh, G. N., Horne, R. A., and Channing, D. M. (1987). A study of telephone advice in managing out-of-hours calls. *J. Roy. Coll. Gen. Pract.*, **37**, 301–4.

Appendix 3: Answering machines, diverters, and pagers

(Prices quoted are those applicable in 1988.)

Answering machines

There are over 200 different models currently available. As one example, the Betacom LR3 Answering Machine can be purchased for £55.95, and a special 2-way adaptor is also required at an extra cost of £3.99. A relatively inexpensive BT model can be purchased for about £80. A more expensive model such as the Challenger (approx. £250) allows up to three minutes for outgoing announcements: replaying of messages is activated by a special voice code from any telephone. It can also page the doctor over a wide area, whenever a call comes in.

The reader is referred to the section on maintenance (p. 14).

Pagers

The range of this equipment has been indicated (p. 13). Most general practitioner needs are fully met with simpler models such as the BT Tone pager. The initial charge is £20, with a monthly rental of £11. If the subscriber is prepared to pay an initial charge of £110, the rental falls to £7 per month.

Diversions (see p. 11)

(a) Temporary transfer through the change number inter-cept (CNI) system is available to the regular user at a charge of £37 per quarter, with an additional charge of 60p per call. For the casual user, the charge is £1.15 per day, but there is a minimum charge of £5.75.

(b) Subscriber-controlled transfer (SCT) diverts calls to the duty doctor's number provided it is within the exchange area. An installation charge of £22 is made for a single alternative number, and rental is £37 per quarter. A group of numbers can be integrated into the system for an installation charge of £55.

Customer-controlled forwarding (CCF), with automatic interception and diversion at the central exchange, can relay calls to a variety of pre-programmed numbers, with the facility of controlling the diversion from the doctor's own telephone equipment. The installation charge is £100, and the rental £60 per quarter. CCF combined with an answering service remote from the surgery premises (for example, Aircall) can relieve the doctor's spouse of the burden of phone sitting (see p. 17). Charges for such services are relatively high—about £250 per quarter.

Appendix 4: Educational exercises

The following six scenarios, based on actual experiences, are designed to allow the reader to apply to patient care some of the concepts discussed in this booklet. To get the most out of this section the reader is invited to commit responses to paper before turning to the discussion on pp. 61 *et seq.*

Telephone call No. 1

The coughing child

Circumstances:	Doctor is on call for a rota of three practices.
Time:	1 a.m. on a winter morning.
Message:	'Please could the doctor come to Suzanne? She can't seem to get breath and has an awful cough.'
Additional information:	Caller is a mother of a three year old, both patients of another practice. Child can be heard, distressed and with stridor, in the background.

(a) What is the likely diagnosis?
(b) What are the main management decisions and likely reasons for them?

Telephone call No. 2

'I don't like his colour.'

Circumstances:	Doctor's night off: has just returned home from an evening with friends.

Time:	11.30 p.m. one autumn evening.
Message:	'Sorry to be ringing you at home at this time of night doctor, but I don't like his colour.'
Additional information:	Caller is the wife of your patient, who is terminally ill at home with lung cancer.

How might you react and why?

Telephone call No. 3

Diversion trouble

Circumstances:	Doctor is about to take over on-call duties for the three practices in the rota.
Time:	6.15 p.m. on Friday evening.
Message:	'I can't get the yellow practice phones through: the others seem OK.'
Additional information:	The receptionist is fully conversant with the SCT system which combines all three practice lines, and automatically diverts calls to the doctor's house within the same exchange area. The practice has recently opted in to the British Telecom Total Care maintenance system. The on-call doctor has just returned home.

What action might you take in these circumstances?

Telephone call No. 4

Priorities

Circumstances:	The doctor is on-call for a large group practice of 22 000 patients.
Time:	Midnight on June evening.

Appendix 5:   Discussion on points raised by the exercises

Should the reader's reactions to those scenarios differ from what follows, he or she might like to consider the reasons for any differences.

The coughing child

Laryngitis stridulosa ('croup') is a likely diagnosis.

A visit is indicated to confirm the diagnosis and, if appropriate, to reassure the anxious mother. Before the doctor visits, he might give advice about warmth and humidity of the atmosphere. Sufficient time for effects of these measures to become apparent (say half an hour) should be allowed to elapse. If the diagnosis is confirmed the doctor may have to resist the urge to initiate antibiotic therapy (see p. 43).

Outcome of real situation

The patient had *laryngitis stridulosa* and was sitting up and looking cheerful. Mother was more relaxed. She was invited to phone a progress report to the practice concerned next day, which she did. Suzanne had had a good night, and now appeared to have no more than a slight cold.

'I don't like his colour.'

The doctor appears already to have pledged his willingness to provide care and support whenever requested. So he might wish to respond with a visit promptly (see p. 45).

Outcome of real situation
The doctor did visit immediately, to find that the patient had just died.

Diversion trouble

The doctor might feel it appropriate to share responsibility with the receptionist in this situation by returning to the surgery premises and re-checking the system, and attempting to make a firmer 'diagnosis' before reporting the fault to British Telecom. The fault should be notified to British Telecom and, as a stop-gap, provided the external line system is intact, all practice numbers should be put on to CNI (see p. 12).

Outcome of real situation
There was a fault in the practice switchboard, which was rectified with commendable promptitude by the telephone engineers. The gap was so short that, in the event, recourse to CNI was not required.

Priorities

Among numerous factors, severity of disease applies to both potentially life-threatening situations. In terms of urgency, both are probably true emergencies. The likely outcomes are different, however, with the potential reversibility of obstructive airways disease giving the edge to the asthma patient. Again, a commitment has already been made to visit the first caller. In terms of the intermediary's problems, the 'stroke' patient's son appears to be less able to cope than the more stable wife. It does not appear, from the point of view of driving time, that the 2 visits can be conveniently conflated.

With a rota of the size indicated there should be a contingency plan with a second doctor on call. Failing that, the situation might be dealt with by the doctor attending to the known asthmatic: an ambulance (2-man and with oxygen) may be ordered, and hospital admission arranged by telephone forthwith (p. 36). The way is then open to visit the supposed 'stroke' patient.

Outcome of real situation
The local chest hospital proved fully co-operative and the asthmatic patient was promptly admitted. The 'stroke' turned out to be a transient ischaemic attack, from which the patient was already recovering when seen half an hour later.

'Desperate Dan'

The information given by the colleague alerts the doctor to the possibility of a 'nonsense call'. The state of the caller and the way in which the message has been transmitted turn that possibility into a probability.

The clinical information implies a high probability of serious pathology.

Attitudes to patients of another doctor (whatever the clinical situation) may be different from those a doctor has to those whom he knows. He may also share a feeling of irritation, expressed by many general practitioners, at the prospect of involvement with a household whose members abuse alcohol and drugs.

Can he tolerate a decision to ignore such a call as this?

How might he feel about invoking police protection should he decide to visit—and what are the implications of such a move for doctor–patient relationships in this situation? (see p. 33).

Outcome of real situation
The doctor made a firm decision not to visit and reported accordingly to his colleague next day. Nothing further was heard of this situation.

'She's burning up.'

Three contacts with the medical profession (two of them out-of-hours, all within 24 hours) suggest serious disease, disproportionate parental anxiety, or both. It might be worth-while trying to find out what Joan's mother had gathered from the trainee, and what has been done so far. This probing has to be done in such a way as to avoid giving the mother the impression of the on-call doctor's ignorance, on the one hand, and, on the other, criticism of the trainee or the mother. If a suspicion of over-anxiety is still entertained it might be worth advising the mother that she's not alone in having to cope with this condition, that she could give Joan a tepid sponge-down, that she should continue with medication (if this has been prescribed), and that she should phone back later if she continues to be worried (see p. 35).

Outcome of real situation
The caller contained the situation overnight but put in a further call firmly requesting another home visit at 8.30 a.m. next morning. Joan had no more than a low-grade coryza, and the presentation was only part of a complex family situation.

Index